AN EMERGENCY PLAN THAT COULD SAVE THOUSANDS,

Based on Experiences of Hiroshima and Nagasaki:
Medical Planning, **FDA Scandal, and Soft Targets**

Third Edition

by

Norman Ende, MD, CAPT MC USNR (ret.)
Professor of Pathology & Laboratory Medicine
Department of Pathology and Laboratory Medicine,
Rutgers University,
New Jersey Medical School, Newark, New Jersey, USA

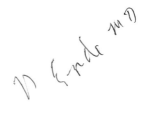

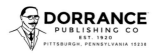

DORRANCE
PUBLISHING CO
EST. 1920
PITTSBURGH, PENNSYLVANIA 15238

Dorrance Publishing Co
585 Alpha Drive
Pittsburgh, PA 15238
Visit our website at *www.dorrancebookstore.com*

ISBN: 978-1-4809-4549-4
eISBN: 978-1-4809-4526-5

CONTENTS

INTRODUCTION

The Food and Drug Administration changed its position on transfusion of unaltered cord blood from an "off-label" product to requiring an investigative new drug permit, affecting multiple diseases and thousands of lives.

For any plan to be successful to save thousands of radiation exposed patients it must address the first 24 hours post-exposures, as this is the most critical treatment period that can greatly improve the odds of survival. Thousands of volunteers will be needed within hours. However, it is not reasonable to expect they will be able to provide the usual "standards of medical care."

A review of the autopsy report of the dead, clinical information obtained from atom bomb survivors, together with our laboratory research, indicates that thousands of victims can be saved in the aftermath of such a catastrophic event based on a workable plan utilizing currently available facilities such as antibiotics, cord blood banks and thousands of volunteers [1-4]. A strong central command, such as the governor or his appointees, with absolute control, is essential.

BACKGROUND

Human umbilical cord blood (HUCB) was given in the U.S. as far back as 1914 [5]. In 1938, Goodall made the following comment about the safety of human umbilical cord blood [6]: "In the many transfusions with cord blood, there has not been one untoward reaction, not a single rise in temperature even to a fraction of a degree." These early studies also indicated that multiple units of cord blood could be given simultaneously, "Two or more fetal bloods may be given simultaneously, necessary after separate matching" [6].

Published in 1972, my brother and I reported that multiple units were given in the first recorded transplant utilizing human umbilical cord blood with minimal immune suppression [7,8]. During that period (1964-1974) 139 ABO compatible fetal cord blood transfusions were given to 15 terminal patients without any adverse reaction [9]. A review of our cases indicated that in addition to the one case reported there were probably several successful transplants.

In 2005, the US Congress established National Cord Blood Depositories (Public Law 109-129) to help restore damage to the bone marrow in case of a nuclear explosion from a terrorist attack or an accident [10]. In 2010, this law was amended to ensure storage of a minimum of 150,000 units [11]. However (to our knowledge) *there is no medical plan in place for utilization of this resource for our civilian population* after a nuclear disaster.

In a nuclear disaster there will be two major components that must be dealt with. First there is **radiation sickness** (nausea, vomiting and diarrhea). This and flash burns will require fluid replacement to prevent dehydration, which should be started within hours. This requires thousands of volunteers to administer fluids.

The second component is **radiation syndrome**. This is due primarily to damage to the immune system (bone marrow) and the intestinal tract.

In case of a nuclear detonation, thousands of patients are likely to suffer from radiation sickness and radiation syndrome.

Medical facilities would be overwhelmed in the first few days after the explosion and unable to perform the necessary laboratory tests to evaluate damage to the bone marrow. ***Prophylactic antibiotic and HUCB transfusions*** should be delivered to large cohorts in the affected areas, based on clinical evidence of radiation sickness. This would greatly enhance the odds of survival.

Critics have stated that this situation may require approval of the FDA to use HUCB as a ***prophylactic measure***; however, it would be expected that Public Law (109-129) (2005) [10,11] would override possible existing restrictions to treat mass casualties after a catastrophic nuclear explosion. In fact, the law was created for this type of emergency. Despite existence of the Law, whenever the necessity of providing cord blood transfusions to hundreds or thousands of radiation victims prophylactically, the FDA objections on cord blood transfusions are always raised. Even though cord blood transfusions have been utilized for over 100 years and are believed to be as safe as or safer than adult donor transfusions (6), the FDA has ruled that transfusion of cord blood, unless utilized as marrow transplantation, requires an Investigational New Drug permit.

In 2002, however, the FDA ruled cord blood transfusions can be utilized as an "off labeled product" (Attachment A), shortly thereafter the FDA made a reversal *ruling that an Investigational New Drug (IND) permit is required. No logical medical reason has been given as*

4

RE Administration of Human Cord Blood into ALS Patients2
From: McNeill, Lorrie [MCNeill@cber.fda.gov]
Sent: Friday, October 25, 2002 2:19 PM
To: 'paul@coqui.net'
Subject: RE: Administration of Human Cord Blood into ALS Patients

Cord blood and hematopoeitic stem cells are the same thing. Cord blood that is
minimally manipulated (meaning it is collected/pooled/stored/tested for infectious
diseases) may be used in the U.S. without prior approval by FDA.
Cord blood that goes through more extensive manipulation (i.e., is processed that
involves adding something to it like a drug, or manipulation of the
cells) may be used only under an investigational new drug application.
Therefore it is not illegal to transfuse product as you have described below, as it
involves only minimal manipulation.

I hope this answers your question. If not, please feel free to contact me again.

Lorrie MCNeill
FDA/CBER

-----Original Message-----
From: Paul Alcalde [mailto:paul@coqui.net]
Sent: Friday, October 25, 2002 1:11 PM
To: MCNeill, Lorrie
Subject: RE: Administration of Human Cord Blood into ALS Patients

Dear Mrs. Harrison:

Does this mean that human Cord blood without hemap. stem cell manipulation can not
be used by any physician in the US. What about the cord blood replacing bone marrow
transplants currently being performed at various Oncology centers for Leukemia is
that Illegal to the FDA ? Since it is blood with idential HLA matching not
differentiated hemap stem cells. There is no manipulation whatsoever in the cord
blood transfussion. We are not talking about the cells manipulated or separated from
the blood, we are talking about the cord blood retrieval pooled as blood itself that
carries high amount of embryonic stem cells neither separated or differentiated into
stem cells. I want to get this concept clear. It is the use of the whole cord blood
not the cells alone, even though it is rich in hematopeitic stem cells.Is this
procedure illegal to perform?
Could you clarify my doubt?

-----Original Message-----
From: MCNeill, Lorrie [mailto:MCNeill@cber.fda.gov]
Sent: Friday, October 25, 2002 12:51 PM
To: 'paul@coqui.net'
Subject: RE: Administration of Human Cord Blood into ALS Patients

Dear Mrs. Alcalde -

Cord blood cells, which are also know as hematopoeitic stem cells, are not subject
to pre-market review and approval by FDA under the agency's current regulations.
What this means is that FDA does not approve cord blood for any particular use. In
the U.S., banks exist that store cord blood for possible future use. These banks are
not currently regulated by FDA, but will be regulated beginning in January 2003. In
January, facilities which collect and store hematopoeitic stem cells (i.e., cord
blood), will be required to register with FDA and follow certain donor eligibility
requirements and Good Tissue Practices (once these regulations are finalized). FDA
would not require a facility (hospital) to submit an investigational new drug
application (IND) for hematopoeitic stem cells, provided the cells are only
minimally manipulated prior to use.

Page 1

ATTACHMENT A

RE Administration of Human Cord Blood into ALS Patients
From: McNeill, Lorrie [McNeill@cber.fda.gov]
Sent: Friday, October 25, 2002 1:51 PM
To: 'paul@coqui.net'
Subject: RE: Administration of Human Cord Blood into ALS Patients

Dear Mrs. Alcalde -

Cord blood cells, which are also know as hematopoeitic stem cells, are not subject to pre-market review and approval by FDA under the agency's current regulations. What this means is that FDA does not approve cord blood for any particular use. In the U.S., banks exist that store cord blood for possible future use. These banks are not currently regulated by FDA, but will be regulated beginning in January 2003. In January, facilities which collect and store hematopoeitic stem cells (i.e., cord blood), will be required to register with FDA and follow certain donor eligibility requirements and Good Tissue Practices (once these regulations are finalized). FDA would not require a facility (hospital) to submit an investigational new drug application (IND) for hematopoeitic stem cells, provided the cells are only minimally manipulated prior to use.

Registration with FDA does not imply that the Agency endorses a particular cord blood bank. What it means is that the facility will be subject to inspection by the Agency to assure compliance with the tissue regulations. More information on these regulations may be found at <http://www.fda.gov/cber/tiss.htm>. In particular, the rule requiring registration may be found at <http://www.fda.gov/cber/rules/frtisreg011901.htm>.

If you have additional questions, please feel free to contact our office again.

Lorrie Harrison McNeill
Director
Division of Communication and Consumer Affairs Center for Biologics Evaluation and Research/FDA phone 301-827-2000/fax 301-827-3843 e-mail mcneill@cber.fda.gov

ATTACHMENT A (CONTINUED)

to why an IND was needed only bureaucratic machinations. Attached is their original ruling and their latter response when we attempted to utilize cord blood to treat the neurological patients injured in the Iraq war {see attachments B,C (page 10),D}. Their final telephone call (no written response) was that an IND permit was required. However, we believe that an executive order in an emergency should overrule the FDA. *An effective plan to save thousands of lives has to be developed months in advance. The country cannot allow, what the military believing is an inevitable event, a nuclear explosion where thousands could be saved be thwarted by the Food and Drug Administration machinations.*

The second major component of dealing with a nuclear explosion is Acute Radiation Syndrome, which will likely require bone marrow

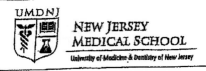

NEW JERSEY
MEDICAL SCHOOL
University of Medicine & Dentistry of New Jersey

May 17, 2006

Director of FDA
Center for Biologics Evaluation and Research
1401 Rockville Pike, Suite 200N
Rockville, MD 20852-1448

Dear Director of FDA

The enclosed documents speak for themselves.

I have never been able to determine the motivation or reasoning behind the FDA's reclassification of cord blood treatment from an off-labeled product to an Investigative New Drug (IND). Is it because of the patent on cord blood? Now that the patent has been nullified in Europe and the US, is the IND still necessary to use cord blood for non hematopoietic diseases such as ALS, Parkinson's, Diabetes I and II, Prostate Cancer, etc.? Or is IRB clearance alone sufficient?

Sincerely,

Norman Ende, M.D.
Department of Pathology
85 So. Orange Avenue
Newark, New Jersey 07103-1709
Phone: (973) 972-6289
Fax: (973) 972-7293

ATTACHMENT B

DEPARTMENT OF HEALTH & HUMAN SERVICES   Public Health Service

Food and Drug Administration
1401 Rockville Pike
Rockville, MD 20852-1448

August 11, 2006

Norman Ende, MD
Dept. of Pathology
185 So. Orange Avenue
NJ Medical School
Newark, NJ 07101

Dear Dr. Ende:

I am writing in response to your recent letters to Acting FDA Commissioner, Dr. Andrew von Eschenbach and to Dr. Jesse Goodman, Director of FDA's Center for Biologics Evaluation and Research (CBER). CBER, one of six centers within FDA, is responsible for the regulation of biologically derived products, including blood and components for transfusion, plasma for further manufacturing and plasma derivatives, vaccines, allergenic extracts, and cellular, tissue and gene therapy products.

In your correspondence about your proposal to treat ALS and type 1 and type 2 diabetes using cord blood, you raise several issues. As to the matter of withdrawn patents referenced in your May 22, 2006 letter, FDA does not issue patents. For matters related to patents, we refer you the United States Patent and Trademark Office (USPTO) for its criteria (http://www.uspto.gov/).

FDA *does* regulate products to protect human health. Specifically, human cells or tissue intended for implantation, transplantation, infusion, or transfer into a human recipient are currently regulated as a human cell, tissue, and cellular and tissue-based product or HCT/P. CBER regulates HCT/Ps under Title 21 of the Code of Federal Regulations (CFR) Parts 1270 and 1271. The term "HCT/P" is defined in 21 CFR 1271.3(d). Some examples of HCT/Ps mentioned in the definition are bone, skin, corneas, ligaments, tendons, dura mater, heart valves, hematopoietic stem/progenitor cells derived from peripheral and cord blood, oocytes and semen. The most recent regulations are in 21 CFR parts 1271 available on the web at:
http://www.access.gpo.gov/nara/cfr/waisidx_05/21cfr1271_05.html. These regulations provide accurate definitions that should prove useful in clearing up any misunderstanding about the terms "non-homologous" and "derived from".

Further, in order for something to be "off-label", it must be first be approved or labeled in some way. This does not apply to the unapproved, experimental therapy you describe.

In your letter, it appears you are interpreting the term "derived from" to mean cord blood hematopoietic progenitor cells extracted from unmanipulated placental\umbilical cord blood by some technical process (manipulation). The term "derived from", in the context of the regulations

ATTACHMENT C

and other cited FDA publications, simply refers to the source of the cell product (namely cord blood, peripheral blood, or bone marrow).

FDA's Compliance Program Guide on HCT/Ps outlines in further detail how establishments and clinical investigators are inspected: http://www.fda.gov/cber/cpg/7341002tis.htm. Please see Attachment I (http://www.fda.gov/cber/cpg/7341002tis.htm#atti) which is specific to hematopoietic stem cells derived from cord blood and peripheral blood. Please refer to the relevant excerpts below:

"NOTE: The regulatory framework for hematopoietic stem/progenitor cells (HPC) derived from peripheral or cord blood is dependent upon whether the product meets the criteria in 21 CFR 1271.10(a), and the intended use (i.e. the recipient) of the product.

- If the stem cell products are intended for unrelated allogeneic use (use in recipients unrelated to the donor), then the stem cell products are regulated under 351 of the PHS Act as drugs, devices and/or biological products, and are not intended for inspectional coverage under this program.

- If the stem cell products are intended for autologous use or for allogeneic use in a first or second degree blood relatives, and meet all of the other criteria in 21 CFR 1271.10(a), then the stem cell products are regulated under section 361 of the PHS Act and are covered under this compliance program.

Many HCT/P establishments that manufacture hematopoietic stem cells derived from peripheral or cord blood, manufacture these products for use in both allogeneic, and autologous, or allogeneic use in first or second-degree blood relatives, i.e. it is common for manufacturers to produce both HPCs regulated solely under PHS Act 361 and HPCs regulated under 351 of the PHS Act."

In your recent conversations with Ms. Deborah Lavoie, Regulatory Project Manager in CBER's Office of Cellular, Tissue and Gene Therapies (OCTGT), she has accurately informed you of the requirement of an investigational new drug application (IND) in order to conduct your experimental studies/therapies. I encourage you to review the regulatory framework summary posted on CBER's website to assist in the process: http://www.fda.gov/cber/genadmin/octgtprocess.htm.

Please be assured that FDA is not obstructing clinical trials. We encourage you submit an IND for review and avail yourself of the avenues available to meet with FDA to assist in preparing your IND submission.

If you would like to schedule a pre-IND telecon with OCTGT to discuss your proposed product and clinical trial please see the "Guidance for Industry: Formal Meetings With Sponsors and Applicants for PDUFA Products" found at: http://www.fda.gov/cber/gdlns/mtpdufa.htm. Your request may be faxed to Ms. Deborah Lavoie at 301-827-5357.

The 2002 email correspondence you cite from Ms. Lorrie Harrison-McNeill, has been taken out of context and does not represent our current thinking about the use of cord blood for treating ALS and diabetes. FDA's regulations of human tissue to include cord blood and peripheral blood have evolved since 1993 when CBER first announced its intent to promulgate these regulations. Again, the newest regulations were implemented on May 25, 2005.

ATTACHMENT C (CONTINUED)

In summary, the treatment of ALS and type 1 and type 2 diabetes with unmanipulated human umbilical cord blood is currently considered nonhomologous use as defined in 21 CFR 1271. therefore, and IND is required as specified in 21 CFR 1271.10 and 1271.20, and must meet th requirements of Part 312 of the IND regulations.

Sincerely,

Adrienne Hornatko-Munoz
Chief, Manufacturers Assistance & Technical
Training Branch (MATTB)
Center for Biologics Evaluation and Research
Food and Drug Administration

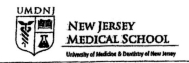

UMDNJ

NEW JERSEY MEDICAL SCHOOL

University of Medicine & Dentistry of New Jersey

D

June 18, 2010
Food and Drug Administration
10903 New Hampshire Ave
Silver Spring, MD 20993-0002

Attn: Deborah Autor, Director of Office Compliance

Dear Deborah Autor,

A few years ago you advised me that cord blood transfusions minimally manipulated (treated as routine blood transfusion) could not be used for neurological diseases, ALS, Huntington disease, neurological trauma, diabetes 1 and 2 etc. without an IND.

We are trying to setup cord blood transfusion for the neurological wounded in Afghanistan and Iraq. As far as we know cord blood transfusion have been safe or safer than adult blood transfusion as far back as 1914 (1) and 1918 (2).

My previous inquiries to you on this matter as to medical use of cord blood transfusion without bone marrow replacement required an IND, but an explanation was not provided by the FDA, only that it was their regulations.

Could you provide this explanation if your restrictions still persist?

We anticipate significant increase in casualties, particularly neurological, in Afghanistan in the near future. We would appreciate a response as soon as possible.

Sincerely,

71. 9 ev6 m' l

Norman Ende, M.D.
Professor of Pathology and Laboratory Medicine
UMDNJ-New Jersey Medical School
Capt, Mc USNR (ret)
185 So. Orange Avenue, MSB C-565
Newark, New Jersey 07101-1709
Phone Office: (973) 972-6289
Fax: (973) 972-7293

References:
1. Rubin, G., *Placenta blood for transfusion*. New York Med J, 1914. **100**: p. 421.
2. Goodall AF, Jr, Altimas, GT & MacPhail, FL. 1938. *An inexhaustible source of blood for transfusion and its preservation*. Surgery, Gynecology and Obstetrics, 66:176-178.

Followed by hard copy via mail

ATTACHMENT D

replacement therapy. Human leukocyte antigen (HLA)-matched bone marrow transplantation might be effective. This, however, would be logistically extremely difficult to utilize in the case of mass casualties. Additionally, the cases reported with adult bone marrow transplants in radiation accidents have had only minimal success [12,13].

A readily available source of stem cells is human umbilical cord blood (HUCB, matched by blood type only (partially HLA matched if feasible), which can potentially restore bone marrow function [14,15]. There are many patients with leukemic bone marrow irradiated and transplanted with human umbilical cord blood [15]. Adult patients usually require 2 or more units to provide the adequate number of stem cells, usually only partially matched for HLA. We are advocating a similar, but an emergency treatment, for tens of thousands of victims of irradiation from a nuclear explosion. The cord blood should be partially matched for HLA if feasible, otherwise only matched for major blood groups.

Pathological Findings
and Laboratory Evidence

Our laboratory results with irradiated mice [14,16-20], together with analysis of the pathology of Hiroshima and Nagasaki victims[2], suggest that many lives could be saved if antibiotics and human umbilical cord blood transfusions are given within the first ~48 hours following exposure to a high dose of radiation [1,20]. This was not available to the patients at the time of the explosion in Hiroshima and Nagasaki in 1945 – neither the broad spectrum antibiotics nor the cord blood banks. The Japanese physicians only had sulfanilamide, which was used in small quanitities.

In animal studies we have noted that transfusion of red cell-depleted mononuclear cells from human cord blood produced not only a transplant chimera but enhanced the recovery of the animals own marrow [21,22]. Cord blood transplantation produces quantitatively less graft versus host disease than bone marrow transplantation, and when it occurs it is less severe than with bone marrow transplants. It is of interest that in our animal studies human cord blood cells given to hundreds of mice have not shown Graft vs Host disease.

Further, we performed a series of experiments with moderately radiosensitive (A/J) mice that were treated with the antibiotic Levaquin and HUCB at different time intervals (24 to 52 hours) after acute whole body lethal exposure of 9 to 10.5 Gy. These results, together with earlier findings from our laboratory [14,16-19], highlight a window of time to effectively treat victims of radiation exposure up to 48+ hours. Theoretically these victims would die if untreated, similar to the thousands (36,000) who succumbed in Hiroshima and Nagasaki in the days after the blasts.

A review of the autopsy reports of the patients that survived the initial blast but died in the next 2 months, bone marrow and intestinal tract showed the classical changes of radiation damage. The pathologists of that time concluded that they could only have saved about 10% of the patients unless the bone marrow was restored [2,3].

DISCUSSION AND MEDICAL PERSPECTIVE

In our experience the concept of trying to establish a medical plan for treatment of mass casualties from a nuclear explosion for the civilian population has been met with extreme resistance at multiple levels, both governmental and academic – locally and nationally. We have been trying to establish a logical plan for over ten years (2003).

Our research started in the early 1990s when we discovered that human umbilical cord blood mononuclear cells could produce significant survival of lethally irradiated mice [14,16]. In 2003, I made contact with General P.K. Carlton, Surgeon General of the Air Force (ret.), and since then we have probed every possible lead to have the United States develop and adopt a medical plan for mass casualties from a nuclear explosion (bomb), not a dirty bomb.

In 2006, as a member of the Society of Medical Consultants to the Armed Services, with Dr. Kenneth Swan, Col MC US Army (ret.), we were able to present this to the military. In 2010, I presented a potential plan in the event of a nuclear attack on the Pentagon, where the population is approximately 20,000. *I received a thank you letter from the Air Force for the nation.* I believe the military has a plan, but it is classified. However, they have repeatedly told me that they *could not produce a civilian plan.* We have continued to attempt to develop a functional medical plan that the state and federal governments will adopt.

Approximately eight years ago we presented this plan to the administration of the city of New York but were unable to obtain any executive attention. We believe that other nations may have plans, but they are classified.

Approximately ten years ago (2006), Dr. Ruifeng Chen, who was a Chinese citizen and had performed many of the studies with me, met with President Hu of China in his pre-promotion trip. He was quite interested and ordered his secretary to take notes. Whether China has a plan, we do not know, but shortly thereafter there was a survey of all the cord blood banks in China.

Several years ago our basic plan was sent to Britain and Israel. I did not hear from the British, but I received a simple thank you note from Israel.

In February 2010 the concept of Mass Casualties Management was presented to the White House National Security staff by General P.K. Carlton, Surgeon General of the Air Force (ret.).

A similar plan was presented to Gov. Christie's Homeland Security for the state of New Jersey on October 3, 2011.

The defining characteristic of a nuclear disaster in comparison to other explosions is that in all other explosions those who walk away having survived the initial blast (walking wounded) will probably live. In a nuclear disaster, however, those that can walk away from the explosion will die by the thousands. But they could be saved.

Currently, there is little or no evidence that a Federal or State Government has an operational plan to deal with the massive number of *civilian casualties* from a nuclear explosion; similar to the casualties that occurred at Hiroshima and Nagasaki. There is significant literature addressed to various aspects of the effect and destruction of a nuclear explosion describing various agencies, support services, committees, resources, and counter measures to assist patients and cities in this type of radiation emergency [12,23,24]. All of these suggested plans, and support systems involve "medical standard of care" which are not likely to be applicable in the scenario of a devastating nuclear explosion involving thousands of exposed patients. It is simply not possible to maintain "standards of care" in this setting.

The devastation of the nuclear bomb explosions in Japan has to be considered as a template for what could occur in a modern American city or metropolis, such as New York. Hiroshima, however, had few concrete and brick buildings. The effects of the blast and flash burns will therefore be considerably different in an American metropolis. On a relative basis, the percentage of blast and burn victims in Hiroshima may have been greater than what would occur in a metropolis. In a metropolis, the blast and heat will be forced upward by tall concrete structures. However, energetic radiation, such as 1 MeVu rays, may penetrate through 1-2 feet-thick concrete. High energy radiation can penetrate 6 feet of concrete. An air-burst over a metropolitan area could produce many more casualties due to the effects of blast, burn, and irradiation depending on the time of day. However, this type of attack is less likely to occur from terrorist activity. Hiroshima and Nagasaki were destroyed by air-burst explosions.

Since radiation sickness can begin soon after irradiation, with nausea, vomiting and diarrhea producing dehydration [25,26], intravenous fluids must be given within 12 to 24 hours, preferably 12 hours, to avoid collapse, dehydration, electrolyte loss and death. Since victims will attempt to walk away from the explosion site, inability to walk and then collapse will occur shortly after the explosion. Similarly, patients with burns will require IV fluid administration. At Hiroshima and Nagasaki, in those victims which survived 20 days, the nausea and vomiting persisted for an average of 2.5 days [4]. Antibiotics must be given as soon as possible to decrease the risk of invasive infection and septicemia [20,25]. Our results indicate that lethally-irradiated animals that were treated with antibiotics alone within 4 hours after irradiation showed significant evidence of increased survival.

In a mass casualty scenario, patients will have varying degrees of radiation dose-dependent damage to the bone marrow and the immune system [25,26]. It must be assumed in this type of emergency, that if these patients present with nausea, vomiting, and diarrhea, the immune system is likely to be compromised [25,26]. If possible, victims with diarrhea should be given priority as a triage strategy. There-

Fig. 1 Hiroshima and Nagasaki Atomic Bomb Casualties

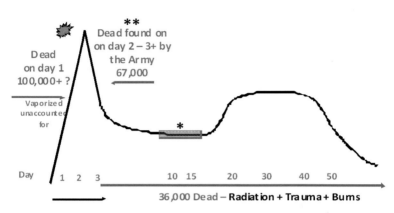

Dead on day 1 100,000+ ?

Vaporized unaccounted for

** Dead found on on day 2 – 3+ by the Army 67,000

*

Day 1 2 3 10 15 20 30 40 50

36,000 Dead – **Radiation + Trauma + Burns**

Walking Wounded - *most of these could be saved*

* Period during which the death rate decreased.

* *Dead found along trails and roads; many showing burns. The combination of radiation sickness and burns lead to rapid dehydration.

Not to Scale Diagram

Fig 2: Time of Death in 757 Fatal Cases

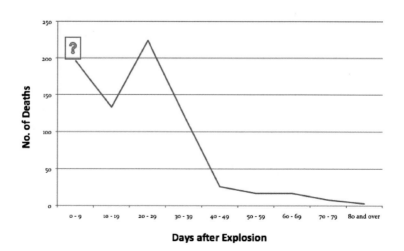

No. of Deaths

Days after Explosion

0 - 9   10 - 19   20 - 29   30 - 39   40 - 49   50 - 59   60 - 69   70 - 79   80 and over

Extrapolated from Table 5.16, Medical effects of the atomic bomb in Japan. Oughterson, A.W. , Warren, S.

fore, protective broad spectrum antibiotics should be administered as soon as possible to these patients to prevent lethal infections [20]. This can be readily accomplished if patients already have intravenous lines for administration of fluids to prevent dehydration. Our recent laboratory findings indicate that early protection, by an antibiotic (Levaquin), of mice that received whole body supra-lethal irradiation, has enabled human cord blood cells to be effective in enhancing survival when administered 24 to 52 hours post-exposure. These findings are consistent with current medical practice. In patients treated with whole body irradiation for hematologic malignancies who receive a transplant for marrow replacement, there is a period of time before the transplanted marrow recovers. These patients are treated prior to radiation therapy or immune therapy with broad-spectrum antibiotics, antifungal and antiviral compounds to avoid infection.

The attempt to negate the value of human cord blood transplants for patients who may receive lethal levels of irradiation from a nuclear explosion, compared to the relative failure of adult bone marrow transplants for lethal irradiation therapy, is unjustified. In an article on contingency planning for a nuclear event in 2008, there were only 31 patients who have undergone allogeneic HSCT (human stem cell transplantation) after accidental radiation exposure [12,13]. *There was only one human umbilical cord blood transplant.* In this report [12], while those receiving human bone marrow had questionable results, the one case at Tokai-Mura, Japan was exceptional. This patient although he had been irradiated with 8-12 Gy over the upper body, had received only one unit of cord blood cells [27]. He lived for 210 days and died from gastrointestinal bleeding and respiratory failure. While children treated for leukemia usually receive only one unit, adults usually require 2 or more units for a successful outcome following marrow ablation. This patient received *only one* partially matched unit of cord blood. He developed *a chimera and his marrow was recovering.* He received a successful skin graft for his burns on his face. The patient developed acute gastric mucosa lesions, severe stomatitis with bleeding ulcerations of the mouth and pharynx. He had no evidence of Graft vs. Host disease. He aspirated purulent exudates and developed methicillin-resistant staphylococcus aureus pneumonia.

From the autopsy report the patient died with organizing pneumonia and diffuse alveolar damage. The anterior surface of the body had degeneration of muscle, and the anterior chest wall "showed brown pigmentation, sclerosis and atrophy" [28,29]. These changes are consistent with radiation burns to the face, neck and anterior thorax, which this patient had received. The most significant finding, however, was the marrow, although still hypoplastic, was recovering and had mixed chimerism (the patient's and the donor's hematopoietic cells).

The patient, although he had been irradiated received anti-thymocyte -globulin, cyclosporine and methylprednisolone usually given to patients as a precondition to transplantation. Rapid autologous hematopoietic recovery, however, was recognized after withdrawal of cyclosporine and methylprednisolone [30]. There is a considerable body of literature indicating that immunosuppression is not needed with cord blood transplantation [31,32]. It is worth noting that in the first cord blood transplants reported in 1972 [7] there was minimal immunosuppression and multiple donor units were used [7,9].

What may be of considerable interest to treating radiation victims is that the patient from Tokai-mura criticality incident had ulcerated intestine even at 6 months after the incident. Our lethally irradiated mice that survived 50+ days with the use of human umbilical cord blood mononucleated cells also had intestinal ulcerations, even though they were gaining weight and behaving in a normal fashion. This would indicate that clinically, patients surviving high dose of irradiation would need prolonged follow-up of their intestinal lesions.

In case of a nuclear explosion, similar to that of Hiroshima and Nagasaki, thousands of first responders (volunteers) would be required to administer care to the victims. The usual first responders (policemen and firemen) would go to the explosion site. The others (volunteers) are likely to be assigned to nearby staging areas close to receiving hospitals that are safe from the radiation hazard. They would be engaged in helping the thousands of victims (*walking wounded*) who show evidence of radiation sickness. The symptoms of patients with radiation sickness can vary between individuals, some can develop nausea, vomiting, and diarrhea within minutes to hours after receiving either sub-lethal or lethal levels of radiation. These survivors (walking wounded) who reach or are carried to designated rescue areas, will require intravenous fluid replacement, preferably within 12 hours after exposure and definitely by 24 hours. In case of large numbers these patients may have to be treated in improvised facilities. *Patients with trauma and/or burns who may also have symptoms of radiation sickness will have to be triaged and decisions made concerning hospitalization vs expectancy.*

The Japanese military that came in a day or more after the explosion was not for rescue but for burial. Location of bodies was not identified.

At Hiroshima a Korean nurse, Nancy (Minami) Cantwell came into Hiroshima after the military had disposed the dead [33]. She recently contacted some of her surviving friends that had gone into Hiroshima before the military had removed the dead and informed me that victims had collapsed and bodies were present along trails and roads [3,33]. This would be consistent with collapse from a loss of fluids (dehydration). They noted that many showed evidence of burns and suggested they suffered from dehydration [33]. The combination of nausea, vomiting, diarrhea, and burns would rapidly produce dehydration, electrolyte loss and collapse.

We recommend that thousands of patients coming from a nuclear explosion area with nausea/vomiting be considered as having evidence of probable hematopoietic-bone marrow/gastro-intestinal damage, *unless proven otherwise*, and receive antibiotics and 3 units of cord blood cells (if logistically available). From our animal studies, published and unpublished, we have found that a mixture of cells from three donors is clinically more effective than the same number of cells from a single donor [18]. An adult receiving cord blood for transplantation usually requires 2 units.

Children will have unique problems in receiving intravenous fluids. I recommend 2 units, blood type specific, matched for HLA if facilities are available. Unfortunately administrating fluids to young children present *unique problems and without considerable help from the pediatric community, many will die who could be saved.*

FDA AND CORD BLOOD TRANSFUSIONS

There is more than reasonable experimental evidence, obtained from research on preclinical animal models, that human umbilical cord blood transfusions could be beneficial to multiple diseases, specifically neurological injuries and others. Our attempts to provide treatment with cord blood transfusions for the military when they were suffering from heavy casualties in Iraq were unsuccessful. The military apparently needs assurance from the FDA that they will not block attempts to treat neurological injuries with transfusions of cord blood. There were increasing neurological injuries in Afghanistan for which cord blood treatment would likely prove beneficial. (Reddi AS, Ende N, The Use of Human Umbilical Cord Blood for Wound Healing, Burns, and Brain Injury in Combat Zones. *Mi Med*, 2011 Apr; 176 [4]: 361-3)

In 2002, ±, 2 clinicians, one on the West Coast and one in Georgia started clinical trials on patients with Amyotrophic Lateral Sclerosis (Lou Gehrig's Disease) utilizing Human Cord Blood transfusion. These clinicians had ample evidence that transfusion of cord blood was a safe procedure. Publications, as far back as 1914 indicated that the use of cord blood transfusions was safe. More recently thousands of frozen units have been used for bone marrow replacement (hematopoietic malignancies). By 1991 we knew that human umbilical cord blood cells had unique stem cells that could salvage mice from lethal irradiation. These cells were not adult stem cell or embryonic stem cells. To identify them as being unique cells we identified them as "Berashis cells" (beginning cells). By 1999, studies in preclinical animal models, indicated that human umbilical cord blood transfusions could potentially ameliorate various human diseases.

For the clinicians to be certain of their position, the daughter of one of the patients with Lou Gehrig's Disease contacted the FDA and obtained confirmation (Ms. Lorrie McNeil, Director of Communications, 2002) that transfusion of cord blood did not need clearance from the FDA, it was an off-labeled product. (See Attachment A). Somewhat thereafter, the FDA reversed its position and shut down the clinician in Georgia, threatening him with charges of a felony and demanding that clinicians obtain an Investigative New Drug Permit to transfuse Human Umbilical cord blood. The clinician in California, on hearing of this problem in Georgia, also shut down.

One of the patients, Major Michael Donnelly (U.S. Air Force) who had Lou Gehrig's Disease, had received cord blood transfusions from the clinician based in Atlanta. The patient and his family believed Major Donnelly (who wrote a book on his illness) had a brief but definite remission of his illness as a result of the transfusion. Later, Major Donnelly came to us in the hope of obtaining additional treatment with cord blood transfusions. A neurologist and I tried to obtain an Investigative New Drug Permit, initially for 10 patients, but finally decided on one patient, Major Donnelly. We submitted a request for an I.N.D. permit. We were summarily dismissed by a phone call from the FDA with no written response. The patient's family then contacted Senator Lieberman of Connecticut for assistance. The FDA responded to the Senator's initial inquiry; his second communication was ignored. Major Donnelly died June 30, 2006.

In 2006 when our military was taking heavy casualties in Iraq, my colleague and I believed that transfusions of fresh and possible frozen cord blood would be beneficial for neurological casualties. In pursuit of this concept we contacted the FDA (Attachment B). We asked to know if an Investigative New Drug Permit was still demanded to transfuse human umbilical cord blood in clinical studies, particularly for diseases in which research on preclinical animal models had already been successful ("to use cord blood for nonhematopoietic diseases such as ALS, Parkinson's disease, Diabetes 1 and 2, Prostate cancer, etc."). In response, we received a long letter of bureaucratic, legalistic jargon indicating that it would be necessary to obtain an Investigative New Drug Permit for neurological injury and multiple other disorders (Attachment C). *No medical reasons were given.* All medical indications are that cord blood, when properly tested, is medically as safe as a transfusion of blood from an adult donor properly tested and is probably safer.

Cord Blood Therapy Effectively Improves Animal Models of Human Disease

Ende N, Chen R, Reddi AS. Administration of human umbilical cord blood cells delays the onset of **prostate cancer** and increases the lifespan of the TRAMP mouse. Cancer Lett. 2006 Jan 8;231(1):123-8.

Ende N, Ende M, Chen R, Coakley K, Reddi AS. Prevention of **atherosclerosis** in LDL receptor-mutant mice by human umbilical cord blood cells. Res Commun Mol Pathol Pharmacol. 2005;117-118:125-36.

Ende N, Chen R, Reddi AS. Transplantation of human umbilical cord blood cells improves glycemia and glomerular hypertrophy in type 2 diabetic mice (**type 2 diabetes**). Biochem Biophys Res Commun. 2004 Aug 13;321(1):168-71.

Ende N, Chen R, Mack R. NOD/LtJ **type I diabetes** in mice and the effect of stem cells (Berashis) derived from human umbilical cord blood. J Med. 2002;33(1-4):181-7.

Ende N, Chen R. **Parkinson's disease** mice and human umbilical cord blood. J Med. 2002;33(1-4):173-80.

Ende N, Chen R, Ende-Harris D. Human umbilical cord blood cells ameliorate **Alzheimer's disease** in transgenic mice. J Med. 2001;32(3-4):241-7.

Ende N, Chen R. Human umbilical cord blood cells ameliorate **Huntington's disease** in transgenic mice. J Med. 2001;32(3-4):231-40.

Ende N, Weinstein F, Chen R, Ende M. Human umbilical cord blood effect on sod mice (**amyotrophic lateral sclerosis**). Life Sci. 2000 May 26;67(1):53-9.

Ende N, Lu S, Ende M, Giuliani D, Ricafort RJ, Alcid MG, Deladisma MD, Bagtas-Ricafort L. Potential effectiveness of stored cord blood (non-frozen) for emergency use (**nuclear explosion**). J Emerg Med. 1996 Nov-Dec;14(6):673-7.

Ende N, Czarneski J, Raveche E. Effect of human cord blood transfer on survival and disease activity in MRL-lpr/lpr mice (**systemic lupus erythematosus**). Clin Immunol Immunopathol. 1995 May;75(2):190-5

Ende N, Rameshwar P, Ende M. Fetal cord blood's potential for **bone marrow transplantation**. Life Sci. 1989;44(25):1987-90.

Ende N. The Berashis cell: a review--is it similar to the embryonic stem cell? J. Med. 2000;31(3-4):113-30. **Breast Cancer (MMTV neu mice) and Aged Mice (a model of aging, C51BL/6J)**

In 2010, I wrote another letter asking if the FDA was wrong in their assessment of the need of an Investigative New Drug Permit (Attachment D). In response I received a phone call from the FDA. The immediate response was that each of the conditions I stated in my letter ("Neurological Diseases, ALS, Huntington Disease, neurological trauma, diabetes 1 and 2, etc.") would need an I.N.D. In the course of the conversation I explained there was also evidence that human umbilical cord blood cells were beneficial for wound healing. After some further discussion she stated she would call me back. A year elapsed and there was no further response. The immediate question was would the FDA prevent the military from utilizing human cord blood for battlefield neurological injuries (see Military Medicine Vol 176 (4). 361-363 April 2011).

The use of cord blood is as safe or safer than adult blood and has been utilized for almost 100 years. In my opinion, if all the diseases we have noted and others require an Investigative New Drug Permit to receive a cord blood transfusion and cord blood transfusion effectively improves human diseases, we are dealing with a *great medical tragedy and scandal.* It is medically ludicrous to require an Investigative Drug Permit for administering cord blood transfusions.

Ms. Lorrie McNeil should be awarded a medal for her interpretation of the FDA regulations and the bureaucrats who reversed her logical medical interpretation and have stubbornly maintained their ridiculous position should be investigated. This matter that has involved thousands of patients should be fully scrutinized and corrected.

We have tried to set up clinical trials in five different countries (China 6x, Poland, Philippines, India and Chile). They always come back with "why can't you set up trials in the USA?" They initially were very interested.

Summary and Conclusion

In most disasters, there is a reasonable chance that existing emergency plans will provide means of survival to those who remain alive following the initial cataclysmic event. When Hiroshima and Nagasaki were destroyed, facilities that we now have, such as broad spectrum antibiotics and human cord blood banks, did not exist. *Consequently, thousands (walking wounded) died days after the blast.*

Currently, there is no evidence that State or Federal Governments have adopted a plan to utilize the aforementioned facilities to save lives in case of a nuclear terrorist attack. This deficiency exists despite the fact that National Cord Blood Depositories were created for this specific goal for treating victims of a nuclear explosion from a terrorist attack in 2005 (Public Law 109-129) [10,11]. Depending on absorbed radiation dose, the victims of a nuclear explosion will likely suffer from nausea, vomiting, and diarrhea, which lead to rapid dehydration and death in the absence of early fluid and electrolyte replacement. Patients with burns also require fluid replacement. They may also suffer varying degrees of injury to the immune system, as was observed in the fatalities at Hiroshima and Nagasaki.

If a "magic bullet" that can restore the bone marrow is discovered by the time we have our first nuclear explosion (which the military believe is inevitable), the clinicians should use it.

If we do not have the "magic bullet or bullets" for recovering the bone marrow, then the cord blood banks that Congress has made available and paid for should be utilized. The effectiveness of the prophylactic use of cord blood can only be evaluated after the disaster. From all the current evidence we have it will do little or no harm and probably save many lives.

In a terrorist nuclear attack thousands of volunteers will be needed. It would be necessary that intravenous fluids be initiated within hours; otherwise there will be few survivors for later treatment. Antibiotics must be given as soon as possible, and cord blood transfusions started early, probably within 48-72 hours following exposure to lethal doses of ionizing radiation. The outcome is likely to promote recovery of the immune system and gastro-intestinal function, which would greatly enhance human survival.

Footnote to history: In the first patient with a successful cord blood transplant, which we reported in 1972, the patient was in Petersburg, VA, and the lab work was performed at Grady Memorial hospital, Atlanta, GA. A shipment of cord blood samples packed on ice from Virginia did not arrive as scheduled. I called Petersburg, VA, and Ms. Marjorie Wood, one of my brother's staff, drove from Petersburg, VA, to the airfield in Richmond, VA, found the package on the tarmac and put it on the next flight. It arrived at Grady Memorial hospital in Atlanta intact.

*The term "magical bullet" or "magische Kugel" was coined by Paul Ehrlich (1854 –1915)

Useful Items for Mass Casualties from a Nuclear Explosion, provided by graduate students and staff of Radiobiology

1) Patients may begin to collapse on the way to the recovery site. First responders will probably have to go forward to meet and assist the walking wounded or treat them with IV fluids where they have collapsed.
2) Nearby first responders should come by bicycle or motorcycle to recovery centers to prevent traffic jams.
3) The bicyclists and motorcyclists should bring bottles of water from home if they have them available.
4) When drones are developed they can deliver supplies of antibiotics and fluids rapidly.
5) Surgical clinics can provide portions of their reserve fluids and antibiotics to assist in case of mass casualties from a nuclear explosion.
6) Pharmacies should have a similar plan as the surgery clinics for providing a portion of their stock to be available for mass casualties ("walking wounded").
7) Fire departments throughout the state should have a plan for decontamination of mass casualties from a nuclear explosion.
8) Anesthesiologists can perform 20-30 IV per hour if the patients are prepared.
9) First responders can have Geiger counters connected to their iPhone and monitor themselves.

SOFT TARGETS AND ADDENDUM

The letter (June 18, 2010) requesting clearance by the FDA for the use of cord blood for various diseases and specifically for the neurological injuries in the war in Afghanistan and Iraq was never fully answered. After an initial call from the FDA, they failed to follow up on my request about the wounded.

In December 2015, the chancellor of Rutgers decided to support the concept for New Jersey, Rutgers New Jersey Medical School and the University Hospital to be the first to develop an operational plan for patient survival from a nuclear explosion and a model for other states to follow.

Since there has been continuous concern about the FDA requirements for an Investigational New Drug application regarding the use of cord blood transfusions for radiation victims and various diseases, the attached letter was sent to the FDA on April 6, 2016. As of January 2017, a reply from the FDA has not been received. (E)

In the last year terrorists have attacked soft targets. This has essentially turned the attacks into battlefield situations where the cause of death is primarily hemorrhage. In such a situation, time is critical for survival. If the program for survival from a nuclear explosion is operational, there would be nearby volunteer help. They would be advised by a central command (Governor's office) to rush to the scene to assist in the emergency to help *stop the bleeding* and to transport the victims to a designated hospital. Other disasters could be helped by these volunteers and a central command.

Most veterans from the current war have had First Aid training and could serve as a nidus for the large number of volunteers needed.

There have been several news releases indicating that placenta derived cells (cord blood comes from the placenta or derivatives from cord blood or placenta) are **undergoing clinical trials in Israel and South Korea on ALS (Lou Gehrig's Disease), Parkinson's Disease, Alzheimer's Disease, and the treatment of mass casualties from a nuclear explosion, suggesting positive results.**

On April 27, 2017 the journal Nature carried the following article "Human umbilical cord plasma proteins revitalize hippocampal function in aged mice (Joseph M. Castellazno et. Al. Nature Vol 544). The author stated "Here we show that human cord blood plasma treatment revitalizes the hippocampus and improves cognitive function in aged mice." The article also states "Our findings reveal that human cord plasma contains plasticity-enhancing proteins of high translational value for targeting ageing-or disease-associated hippocampal dysfunction." The article also states "Cord-plasma-enriched CSF2 improved hippocampal-dependent memory in aged mice, consistent with previous work in aged mice that develop Alzheimer's disease pathology and…"

In the later days of President Reagan's illness with Alzheimer's disease, I sent Nancy Reagan a letter suggesting that the President be treated with transfusions of cord blood for his Alzheimer's disease and enclosed a copy of our article, "HUMAN UMBILICAL CORD BLOOD CELLS AMELIORATE ALZHEIMER'S DISEASE IN TRANSGENIC MICE, A BREIF REPORT." She was gracious enough to answer me and thanked me but stated they were happy with President Regan's treatment. Our Alzheimer's survival study was on mice developed by Karen Hsiao, M.D., Ph.D. [TG(HuAPP 695.SWE)2576]. These mice had a p-value of 0.001 meaning the study treatment had statistically significant results (Journal of Medicine Vol. 32, NOS. 3&4, 2001).

In our ageing studies the mice were C5BL/6J. The increase of their life span had a p-value of 0.0267 again signifying statistically significant results (THE BERASHIS CELL: A REVIEW, IS IT SIMILAR TO THE EMRYONIC STEM CELL? Journal of Medicine Vol. 3, NOS 3&4, 2000).

Human umbilical cord blood cells were used over 16 years ago to treat various mice models. The Food and Drug Administration scandal of demanding an Investigative New Drug Permit without a medical reason is an outrage (Attachment C, page 10). *The delay of clinical trials has potentially cost thousands of life years.*

ATTACHMENT E

The Food and Drug Administration's Commissioner   April 6, 2016
U.S. Food and Drug Administration
10903 New Hampshire Avenue
Silver Spring, MD 20993-0002

Dear Dr. Califf,

   We are attempting to have the state of New Jersey prepare and have an operational plan to treat mass casualties from a nuclear explosion (1). We know that cord blood transfusions have been given for over 100 years and are as safe or safer than blood transfusions from an adult donor. The FDA has restricted the transfusions of cord blood by the definition of "homologous", not on the safety of the transfusions.

   In view of the FDA restrictive policy (2) about the use of cord blood transfusions, I have to ask the following questions:

1. If a nuclear explosion occurs, during the time New Jersey is developing a functional medical plan for the treatment of the casualties, do the physicians who know of the potential use of cord blood transfusions (1) and administer cord blood; will they face felony charges if they do not have an IND permit?

2. Since we are trying to have New Jersey be the first state to have a functional plan (1), will the state of New Jersey need an IND permit before they make the plan functional?

3. Many of the injured may be given prophylactic cord blood transfusions depending on location of patients, limited clinical findings, such as only nausea etc., and patients with other diseases for which the FDA has demanded an IND permit (2) prior to receiving a cord blood transfusion. Will they be excluded from treatment with cord blood transfusions?

In 2005 the US Congress established National Cord Blood Depositories (Govtrack. US. H.R. 2520: Stem Cell Therapeutic and Research Act of 2005, Public Law 109-129. 2005.) to help restore damage to the bone marrow in case of a nuclear explosion from a terrorist attack or an accident. In 2010, this law was amended to ensure storage of a minimum of 150,000 units (Govtrack. US. H.R. 6083 - Stem Cell Therapeutic Research Reauthorization Act of 2010. To amend the Stem Cell Therapeutic and Research Act of 2005. 2010).

Would the cord blood banks be penalized or not allow the physicians to give the cord blood transfusions if they did not have an IND permit?

Norman Ende, MD

Professor of Pathology and Laboratory Medicine
Capt, MC USNR (ret)
Medical Science Building, C-565
New Jersey Medical School, Rutgers, The State University of New Jersey
185 South Orange Ave. Newark, NJ, 07103
Phone Office: (973) 972-6289;
Phone Lab: (973) 972-4792
Fax: (973) 972-7493

References:

1. Ende, N. An Emergency Plan that could Save Thousands: Based on Experiences of Hiroshima and Nagasaki. 2nd edition: New Medical Planning Manual. Published on Amazon.com, 2014

2. FDA letter, August 2006.

CC: Wall Street Journal, Congressman Smith, Governor Christie, Senator Menendez, Senator Booker, Steve Andreassen Chief of Staff Chancellor's office Rutgers University.

ACKNOWLEDGMENTS

Through this long struggle I would like to acknowledge my late wife, Beatrice Starr Ende, who always supported my research, even though there was little economic gain. I wish to thank my late brother, Dr. Milton Ende, who gave the first cord blood transplantation to his patients [7] and who energetically supported and provided most of the funds for research on the treatment of mass casualties from a nuclear disaster with human umbilical cord blood. I also wish to thank his staff who helped collect cord blood for his patients and others, who sent specimens to me.

I would like to acknowledge those who helped to create this manuscript. General P.K. Carlton, Surgeon General of the Air Force (ret.). Dr. Edouard Azzam, Professor of Radiology, UMDNJ-NJMS. Kenneth Swan, MD, Professor of Surgery (deceased), UMDNJ-NJMS, Donald T. Allegra, MD, Manoosher Khorsidi, MD, Olga Kovalenko, MD, PhD, David Ende, MD, Ruifeng Chen, MD.

In addition, I would like to thank the obstetric physicians and staff of the South Side Regional Medical Center, Petersburg, VA. Lesslie Iffy, MD, Director of Obstetrics and staff at University Hospital, UMDNJ-NJMS, and Celgene who helped provide human umbilical cord blood. I would like to thank the multiple colleagues, students, graduate students, fellows, and postdoctoral fellows, who participated in this research over many years, who are named in the references.

At times when few would believe our findings there were several strong supporters: Dr. Romeo Cabalas, Gen. P.K. Carlton, Surgeon General of the Air Force (ret.), Dr. Kenneth Swan, Professor of Surgery, COL USA (ret.), Dr. Alluru Reddi, Professor of Medicine and Dr. Edouard Azzam, PhD, Professor of Radiology, Dr. Robert Shwartz, Professor of Dermatology, whose support I greatly appreciate.

References

[1] Ende N, Azzam EI. Consideration for the treatment of mass casualties based on pathology of the fatalities of Hiroshima and Nagasaki. Int J Radiat Biol 2011;87 (4):443-4.

[2] Liebow AA, Warren S, DeCoursey E. Pathology of atomic bomb casualties. The American Journal of Pathology 1949;XXV (5):853-1027.

[3] Pellegrino C, editor. The Last Train From Hiroshima: The Survivors Look Back. New York, NY: John MacRae Books, 2010.

[4] Oughterson AW, Warren S, editors. Medical effects of the atomic bomb in Japan (National nuclear energy series. Manhattan Project Technical Section. Division VIII, v.8). New York, NY: McGraw-Hill, 1956.

[5] Rubin G. Placenta Blood for Transfusion. New York, Medical Journal 1914;100:421.

[6] Goodall JR AF, Altimas GT, MacPhail FL. An inexhaustible source of blood for transfusion and its preservation. Surgery, Gynecology and Obstetrics 1938;66:176-8.

[7] Ende M, Ende N. Hematopoietic transplantation by means of fetal (cord) blood. A new method. Va Med Mon (1918) 1972;99 (3):276-80.

[8] Glasser L. The Ende brothers and the arcane history of the first umbilical cord blood hematopoietic stem cell transplant. Transfusion 2009;49 (9):2010.

[9] Ende M. History of umbilical cord blood transplantation. Lancet 1995;346 (8983):1161.

[10] Govtrack.US. H.R. 2520: Stem Cell Therapeutic and Research Act of 2005, Public Law 109-129. 2005.

[11] Govtrack. US. H.R. 6083 - Stem Cell Therapeutic Research Reauthorization Act of 2010. To amend the Stem Cell Therapeutic and Research Act of 2005. 2010.

[12] Weinstock DM, Case C, Jr., Bader JL, Chao NJ, Coleman CN, Hatchett RJ, Weisdorf DJ, Confer DL. Radiologic and nuclear events: contingency planning for hematologists/oncologists. Blood 2008;111 (12):5440-5.

[13] Dainiak N, Ricks RC. The evolving role of haematopoietic cell transplantation in radiation injury: potentials and limitations. BJR Suppl 2005;27:169-74.

[14] Ende N, Ponzio NM, Athwal RS, Ende M, Giuliani DC. Murine survival of lethal irradiation with the use of human umbilical cord blood. Life Sci 1992;51 (16):1249-53.

[15] Chao NJ, Emerson SG, Weinberg KI. Stem cell transplantation (cord blood transplants). Hematology Am Soc Hematol Educ Program 2004:354-71.

[16] Ende N, Lu S, Ende M, Giuliani D, Ricafort RJ, Alcid MG, Deladisma MD, Bagtas-Ricafort L. Potential effectiveness of stored cord blood (non-frozen) for emergency use. J Emerg Med 1996;14 (6):673-7.

[17] Azzam EI, Yang Z, Li M, Kim S, Kovalenko OA, Khorshidi M, Ende N. The effect of human cord blood therapy on the intestinal tract of lethally irradiated mice: possible use for mass casualties. Int J Radiat Biol 2010;86 (6):467-75.

[18] Ende N, Lu S, Alcid MG, Chen R, Mack R. Pooled umbilical cord blood as a possible universal donor for marrow reconstitution and use in nuclear accidents. Life Sci 2001;69 (13):1531-9.

[19] Ende N, Ponzio NM, Giuliani D, Bagga PS, Godyn J, Ende M, Athwal RS. The effect of human cord blood on SJL/J mice after

chemoablation and irradiation and its possible clinical significance. Immunol Invest 1995;24 (6):999-1012.

[20] Ende N, Kovalenko OA, Azzam EI. The necessity of the early use of antibiotics in treatment of mass casualties from ionizing radiation. Int J Radiat Biol 2012;88 (4):381.

[21] Czarneski J, Lin YC, Ende N, Ponzio NM, Raveche E. Effects of cord blood transfer on the hematopoietic recovery following sublethal irradiation in MRL lpr/lpr mice. Proc Soc Exp Biol Med 1999;220 (2):79-87.

[22] Rameshwar P, Smith I, Ende N, Batarseh HE, Ponzio NM. Endogenous hematopoietic reconstitution induced by human umbilical cord blood cells in immunocompromised mice: implications for adoptive therapy. Exp Hematol 1999;27 (1):176-85.

[23] Radiation Injury Treatment Network, Health Resources and Services Administartion, U.S. Department of Helath and Human Services
http://bloodcell.transplant.hrsa.gov/ABOUT/RITN/index.html.

[24] (REAC/TS) REACTS. Guidance for Radiation Accident Management.

[25] Donnelly EH, Nemhauser JB, Smith JM, Kazzi ZN, Farfan EB, Chang AS, Naeem SF. Acute radiation syndrome: assessment and management. South Med J 2010;103 (6):541-6.

[26] Hall EJ, Giaccia AJ. Radiobiology for the Radiologist. Philadelphia Lippincott Williams & Wilkins, 2006.

[27] Nagayama H, Ooi J, Tomonari A, Iseki T, Tojo A, Tani K, Takahashi TA, Yamashita N, Shigetaka A. Severe immune dysfunction after lethal neutron irradiation in a JCO nuclear facility accident victim. Int J Hematol 2002;76 (2):157-64.

[28] Asano S. Multi-organ involvement: lessons from the experience of one victim of the Tokai-mura criticality accident. BJR Suppl 2005;27:9-12.

[29] Uozaki H, Fukayama M, Nakagawa K, Ishikawa T, Misawa S, Doi M, Maekawa K. The pathology of multi-organ involvement: two autopsy cases from the Tokai-mura criticality accident. BJR Suppl 2005;27:13-6.

[30] Nagayama H, Misawa K, Tanaka H, Ooi J, Iseki T, Tojo A, Tani

K, Yamada Y, Kodo H, Takahashi TA, Yamashita N, Shimazaki S, Asano S. Transient hematopoietic stem cell rescue using umbilical cord blood for a lethally irradiated nuclear accident victim. Bone Marrow Transplant 2002;29 (3):197-204.

[31] Riordan NH, Chan K, Marleau AM, Ichim TE. Cord blood in regenerative medicine: do we need immune suppression? J Transl Med 2007;5:8.

[32] Ende N. Our findings conclude that immune suppression is not needed for a successful transplant of cord blood. Journal of Translational Medicine 2007;5 (8).

[33] Cantwell N. A Life in Three Motherlands (Japan, Korea, USA) You Can Do It!! I Did It. New York: Vantage Press, 2006. Personal communications with the author.